Safer Fall

The Possibility is Real

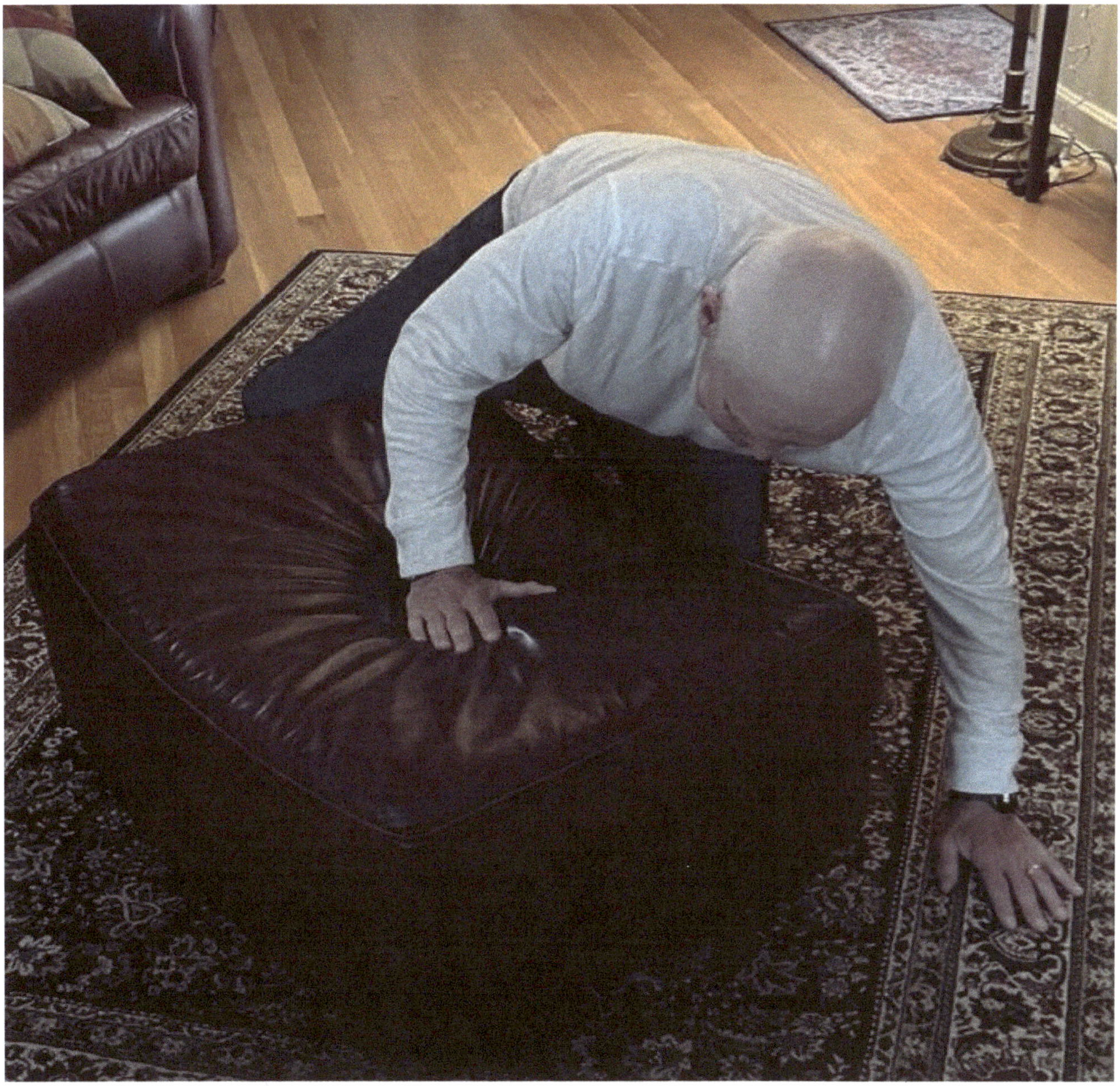

This book is dedicated to the memory of *Paula Schutt.*
Her work to assist others will be an example for us all.

Introduction

The doctor walks into your examination room and softly utters the words that change your life forever. "You have Parkinson's Disease." It all comes together in your mind - all the symptoms you have displayed over time: shaking of the hands; the slow, stiff walk; the poor balance; the lack of facial expressions; difficulty speaking. You are told there are many other symptoms associated with Parkinson's and you can research and prepare yourself for what's to come.

How can you prepare for the uncertain future? How can you prepare for that unknown and that fear? Edmund Burke said "No passion so effectively robs the mind of all its power as fear." We know it is a mistake to give into fear. Making that mistake and learning from it gives us experience. From experience we gain wisdom. This path of learning doesn't have to be walked alone. We can share ideas and concepts with others, thus easing the burden for all.

While the focus of this book is for Parkinson's patients, it is information for everyone, no matter the age or physical condition. It is not *if* we fall but **when** we fall. Can we prepare ourselves for those unexpected moments? The techniques described in this book are not the only methods to fall safer, but are among many other options available. Any method that is used will need effort and training to become comfortable. While watching the techniques being demonstrated is a valuable mental repetition, doing the drills teaches the body and mind to work together. The truth is with each repetition the body finds it is easier to perform the drill.

Before starting any new training, it is wise to consult with your doctor and your caregivers. Having the proper support makes any difficult task easier. Expect to have that fear of getting hurt when starting. Expect the fear of not getting these drills done correctly or easily. Expect the frustration of making a mistake. Then expect the recognition of making a mistake and knowing how to do it better. And doing it better each time.

There are three priorities of *Safer Fall*:

1. Protect the head.
2. Don't try to stop the fall or fight against the energy of the fall.
3. Relax the body and roll. Accept it may hurt (a lot) but the glory (of surviving) lives forever.

The people shown within this book are not models. Some suffer from Parkinson's, others are just old. Physical abilities vary. We feel it is more representative of the people we want to help. We have also increased the size of the font for easier reading. We hope you find value in this book.

It is common sense to take a method and try it, if it fails, admit it frankly and try another. But above all, try something.

\- Theodore Roosevelt

Chapter One: Forward Falls

Kids enjoy slapstick comedy. Someone falling into a mud puddle or doing a header into a pastry table is guaranteed to have them on the floor. As we get a bit older, we may trip walking on an uneven sidewalk. We chuckle to ourselves asking if anyone might have seen us. Then when we are mature, we recognize the dangers of falling and it's not a laughing matter.

Typical Injuries to Avoid

When we fall, our instinct is to stick our arms out to stop the impact or catch something that will slow or stop the fall. The danger in this is exposing our fingers, wrists, elbows and shoulders to painful damage. Imagine a board falling flat on the ground. See the dust kicking up around the board. Now picture a person falling straight-body to the ground with their arms outstretched in front of them. The energy generated from falling at height is enough to break fingers or wrists, dislocate elbows and tear muscles in the shoulders.

Concepts That Protect

One method of falling forward is to land on the forearms which act as a shock absorber for the rest of the body. The head is turned to the side. The danger is the upper arm (triceps) may not be strong enough to stop the falling motion and the body still has direct impact with the ground. The other issue is that if the person forgets to turn their head, the nose smashes on the ground.

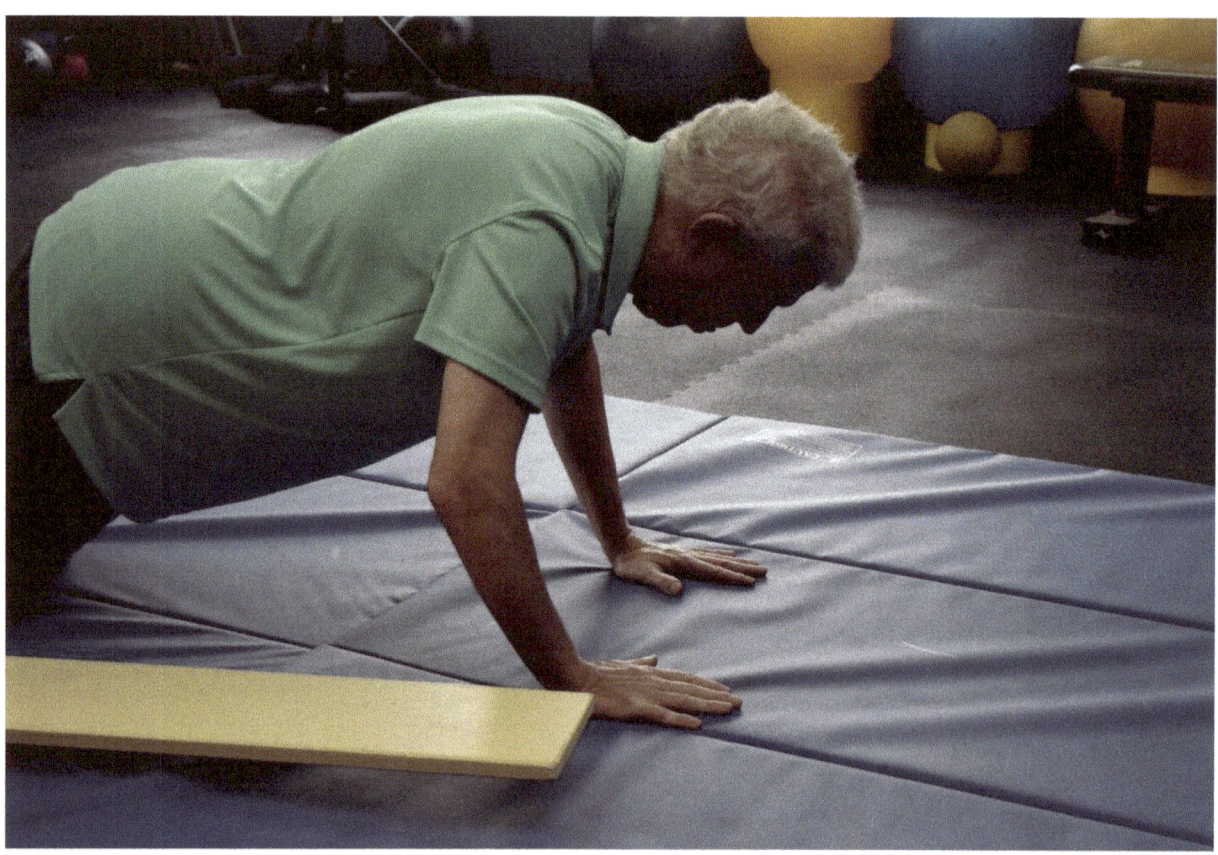

Instead of being a stiff board slapping the floor, imagine a foam roller or a hose bouncing, rolling on the floor. The roller/hose moving in a circular motion eventually stops moving after a while. Falling stiff like a board focuses all the kinetic energy in one spot or area. Falling/moving in a circular motion extends the time to disperse the energy over as large an area of the body as possible. Extending the time of the contact (continuing to roll once on the ground) during the fall will also disperse the kinetic energy.

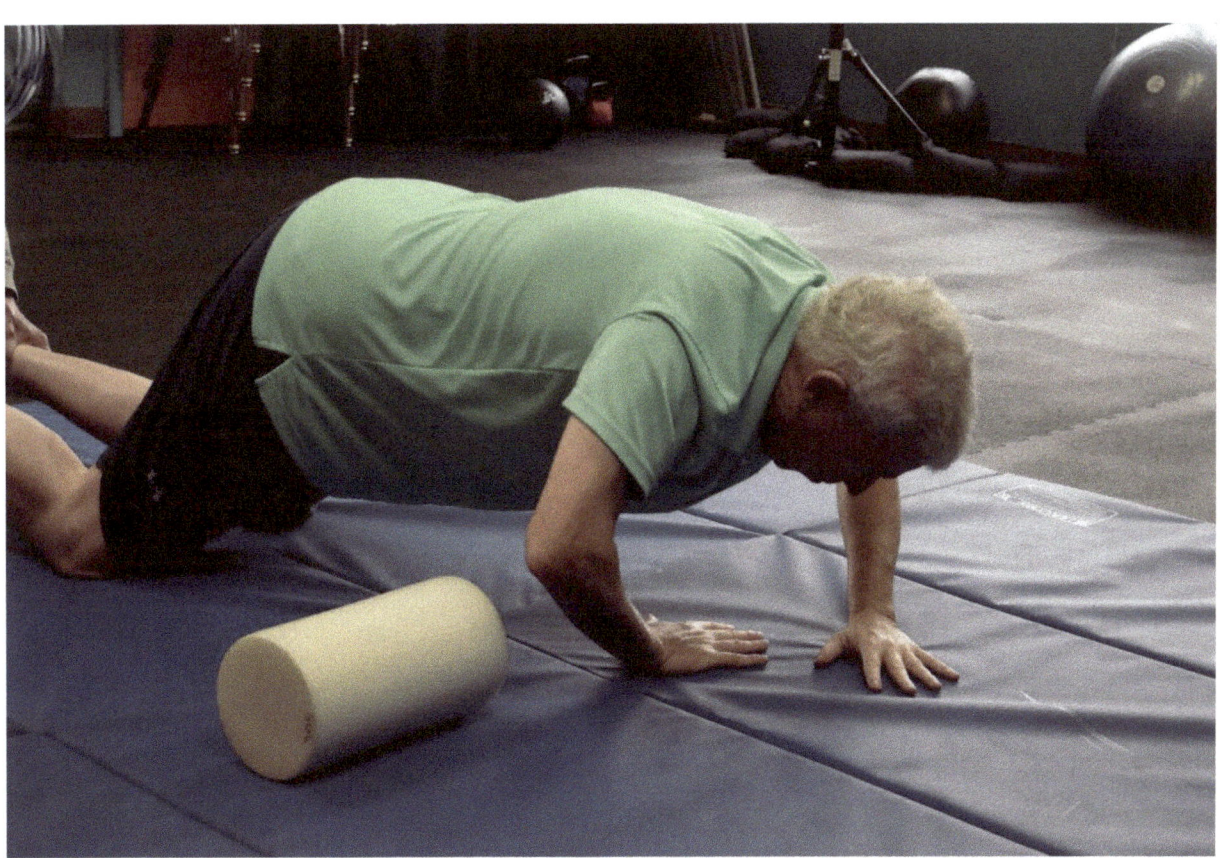

Practice the three priorities of *Safer Fall*:
1. Protect the head.
2. Don't try to stop the fall or fight against the energy of the fall.
3. Relax the body and roll. Accept it may hurt (a lot) but the glory (of surviving) lives forever.

How to Practice

To practice the forward motion roll, we recommend getting an exercise ball and a foam mat if you don't have a nice padded carpet.

Start the drill by laying your chest high on the ball. Falling to the right, place your right hand below your shoulder, bent and searching to find the ground. With the hand towards the centerline of the body, it is in position to start the rolling action. The hand should not try to stop the fall, only to initiate movement towards the elbow and shoulder. The left hand is open and high, above chin level. The left hand is there to protect the head from any hard impacts with the ground. The head is turned away from the fall. This part of the drill requires repetition and training to build muscle memory and confidence. The first priority of a *Safer Fall* is to protect the head by turning the head away from the fall.

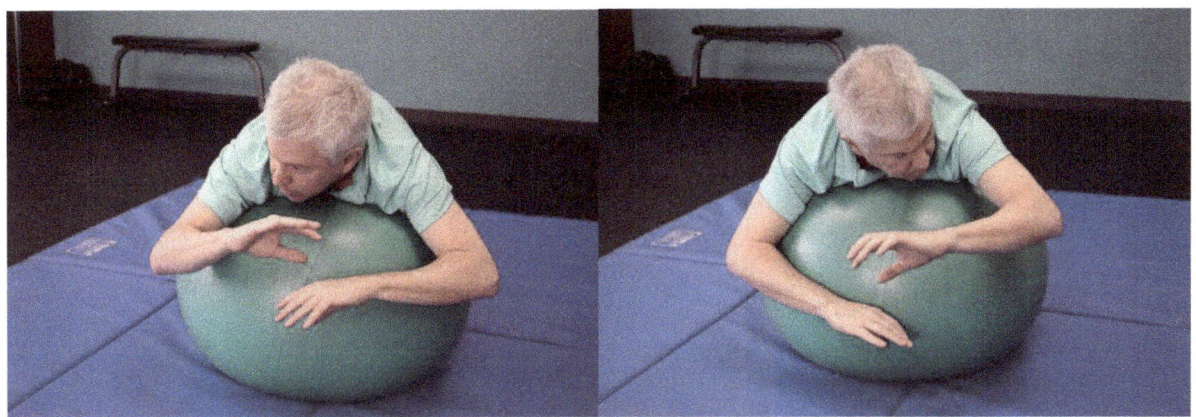

Now we are ready for the second priority of a *Safer Fall*: don't stop/fight the fall, extend the time of the contact during the fall.

With the hands and head in their proper position, push forward and roll over the right shoulder. The right hand typically will hold onto the exercise ball while the left hand braces the head from the ground. Roll until it is comfortable to stop, usually once you are on your back or side. There should not be a lot of noise, no slapping of the mat or floor. If you roll over the shoulder, there will be little noise. If you fall directly to your side (lateral motion), there would be more of a slapping sound. This would be what airborne troops would call landing on the pull-up muscles (abdominal oblique and latissimus dorsi). If you land with a lateral motion, continue to roll. Think of a corkscrew motion, landing on the quadriceps (thighs), then the glutes, the pull-up muscles and if necessary continue to roll to stop once again on the initial fall side. Let the energy dissipate slowly.

Lateral rolls:

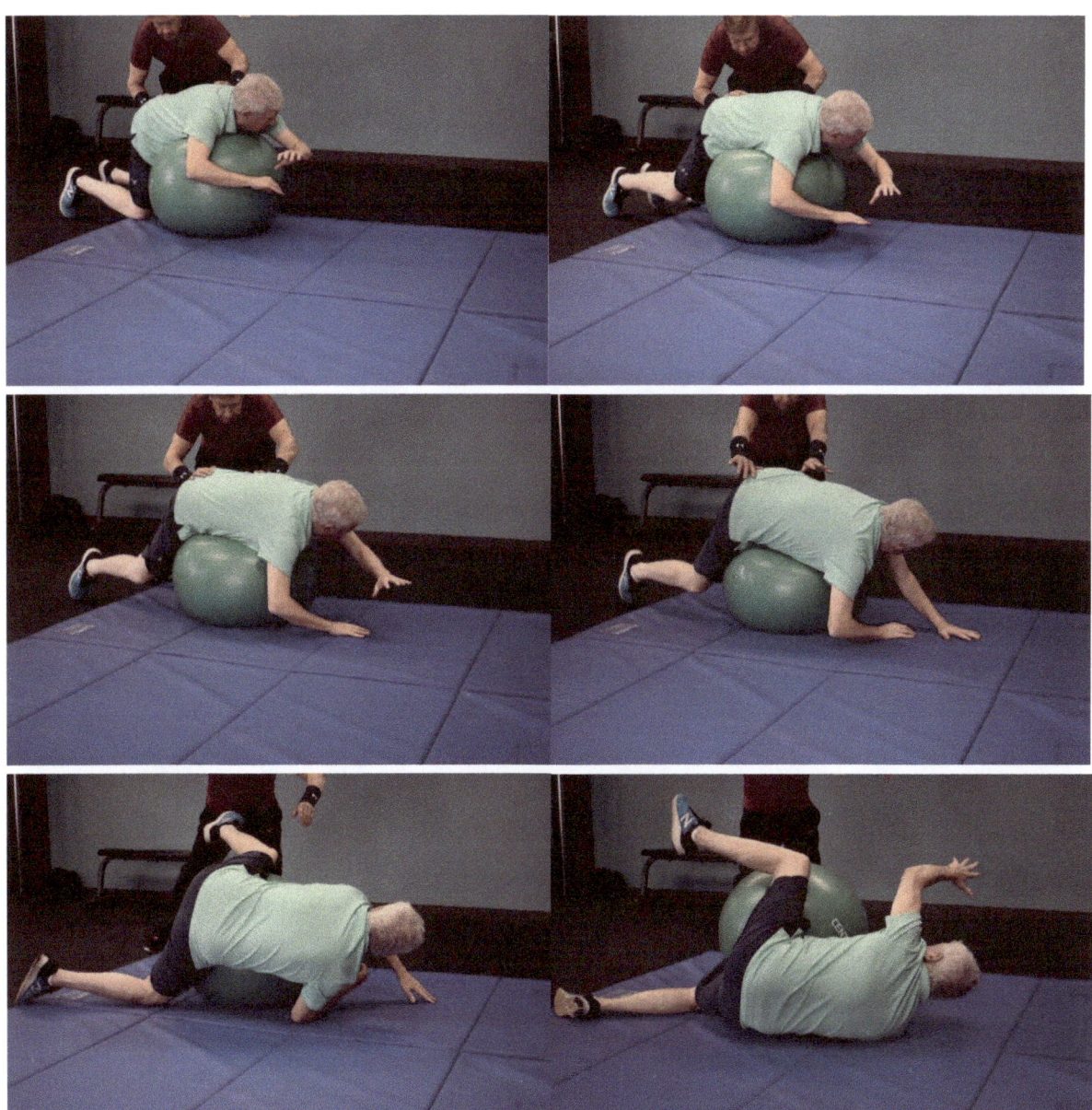

Forward rolls:

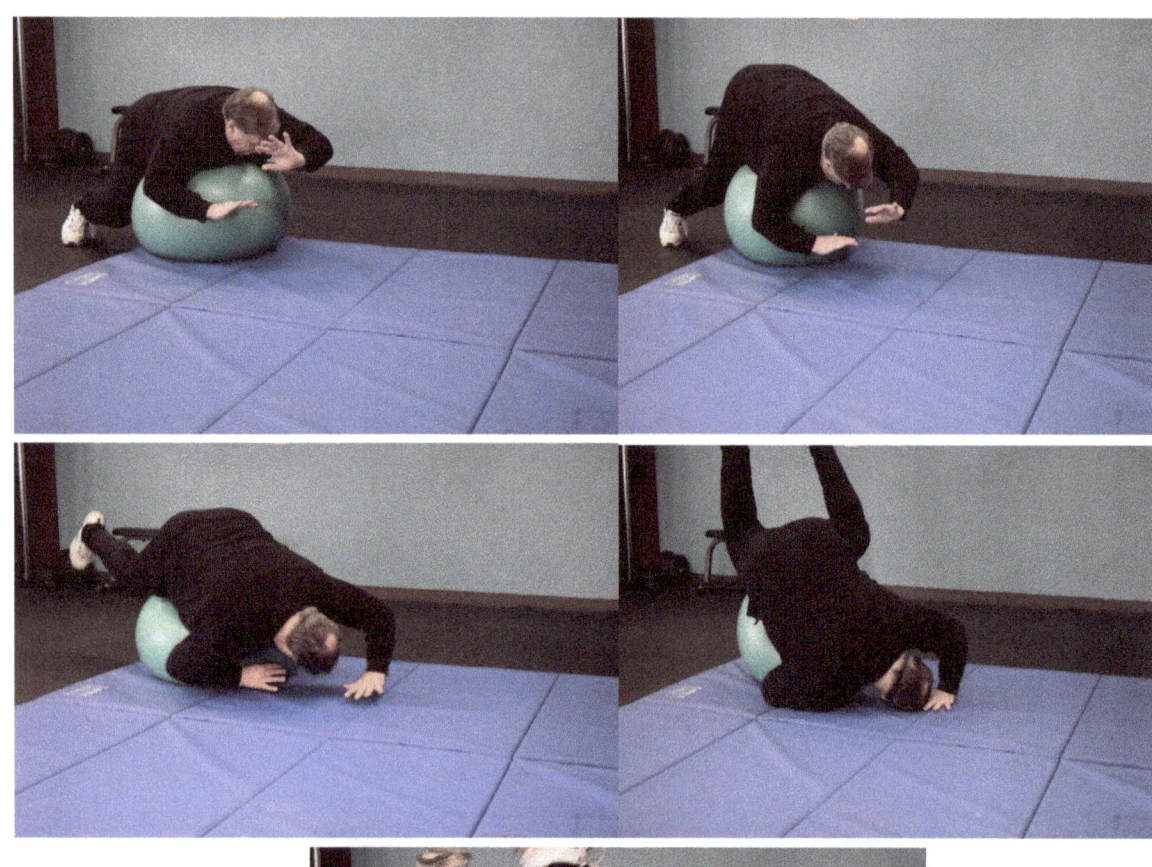

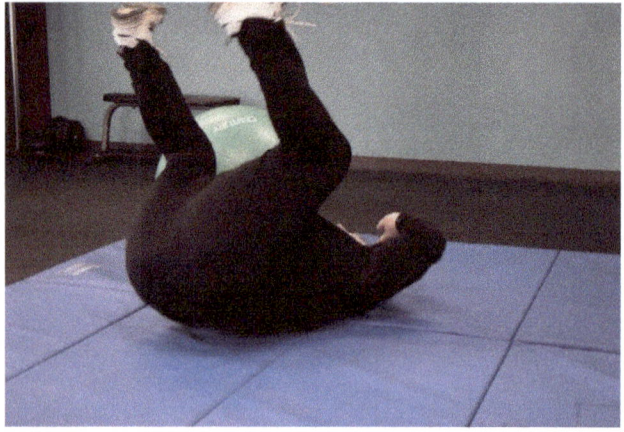

This brings us to the final priority of *Safer Fall*: relax and roll. Accept that it may hurt but glory (survival) lasts forever.

Once on the ground, stop all action and calm yourself. Before moving, do a total body assessment for injury. Start at the head and slowly move down. Shoulders feel in place, allowing arms and fingers to move. Breathe in deeply to see how the ribs feel. Flex the glutes and wiggle the hips to see if there are any problems. Finally, wiggle the toes. Take another couple of deep breaths and attempt to get up, if possible.

After practicing with the ball, attempt the forward roll from a squatting position. The left foot should be slightly in front of the right foot. Get your hands in the proper position and turn the head away. Slowly lean forward to roll over the right shoulder. Let the momentum carry you until you stop.

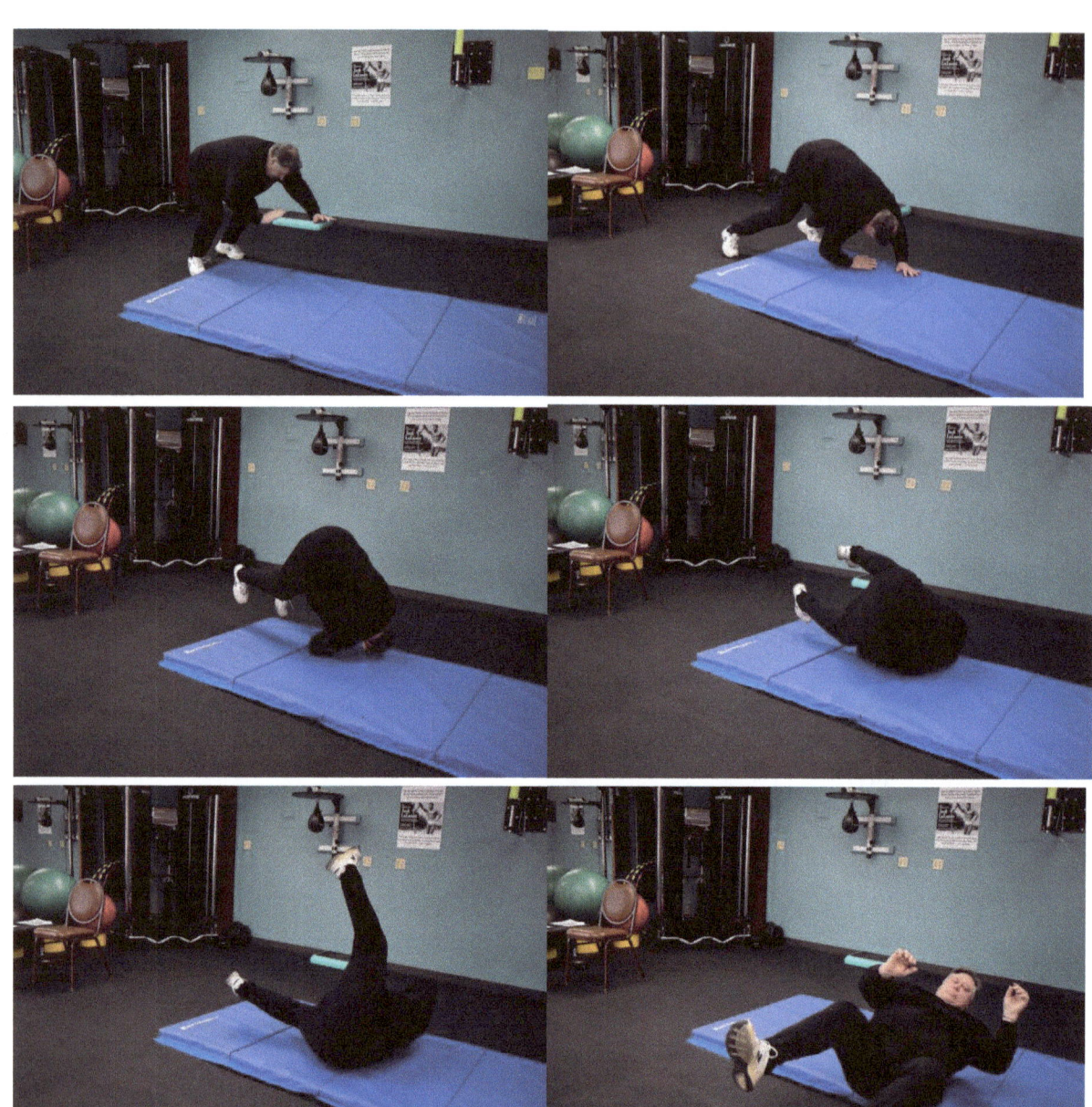

Once you are comfortable falling from a squatting position, practice falling from an upright stance. From the standing position, place your feet closer together, bend the knees slightly, lean forward at the waist, and initiate the roll over the right shoulder. Hand placement remains the same. Stop rolling once the energy dissipates.

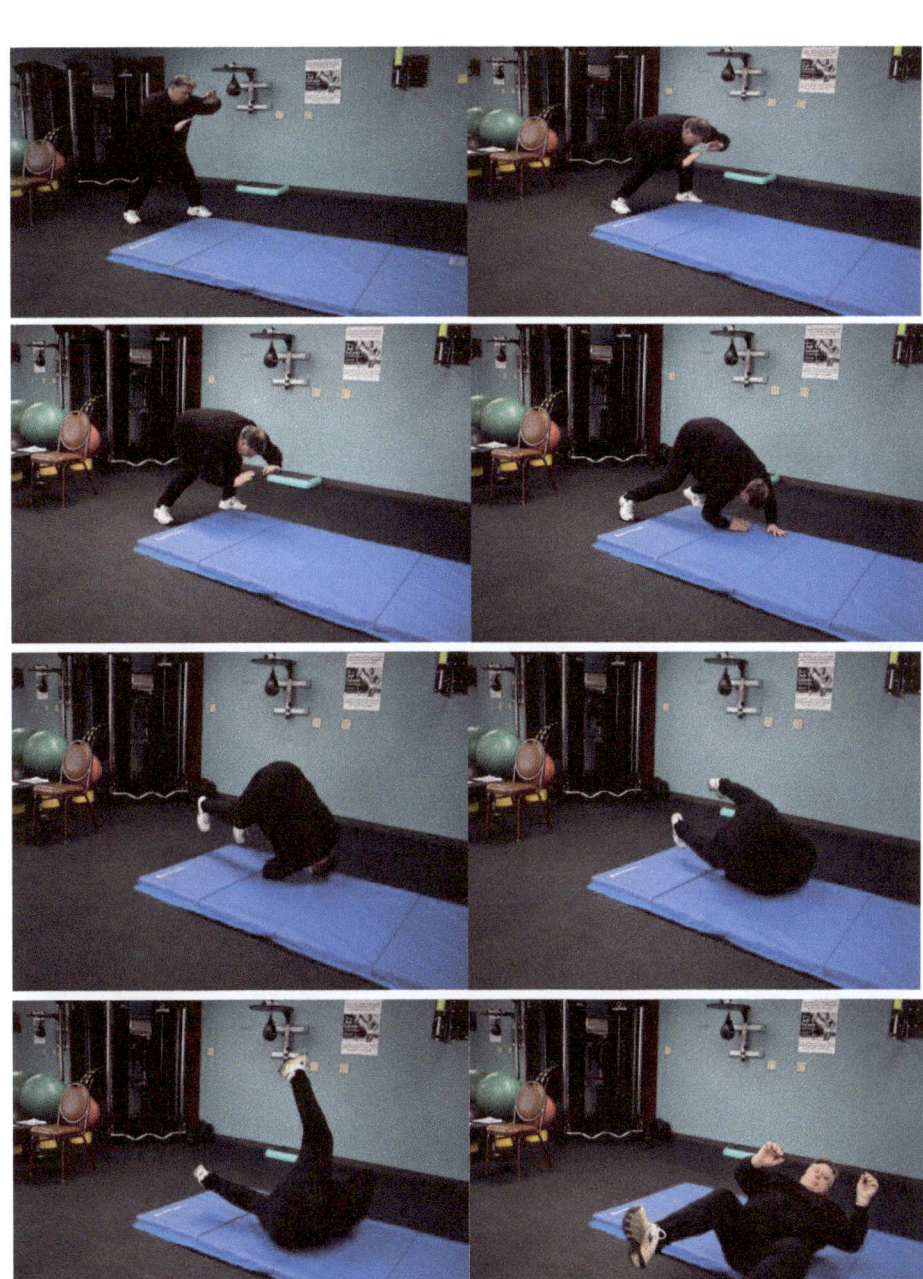

Chapter Two: Backwards Falls

Typical Injuries to Avoid

The fall with the most potential for harm is falling backwards. The arms come out away from the body searching for something to grab hold of while the body stiffens, becoming a board. The body strikes the ground flat with a head snap and bouncing off the ground as force exceeds neck strength. Besides the damage to the head and neck, if the ground is uneven, the force from the fall could damage the spine.

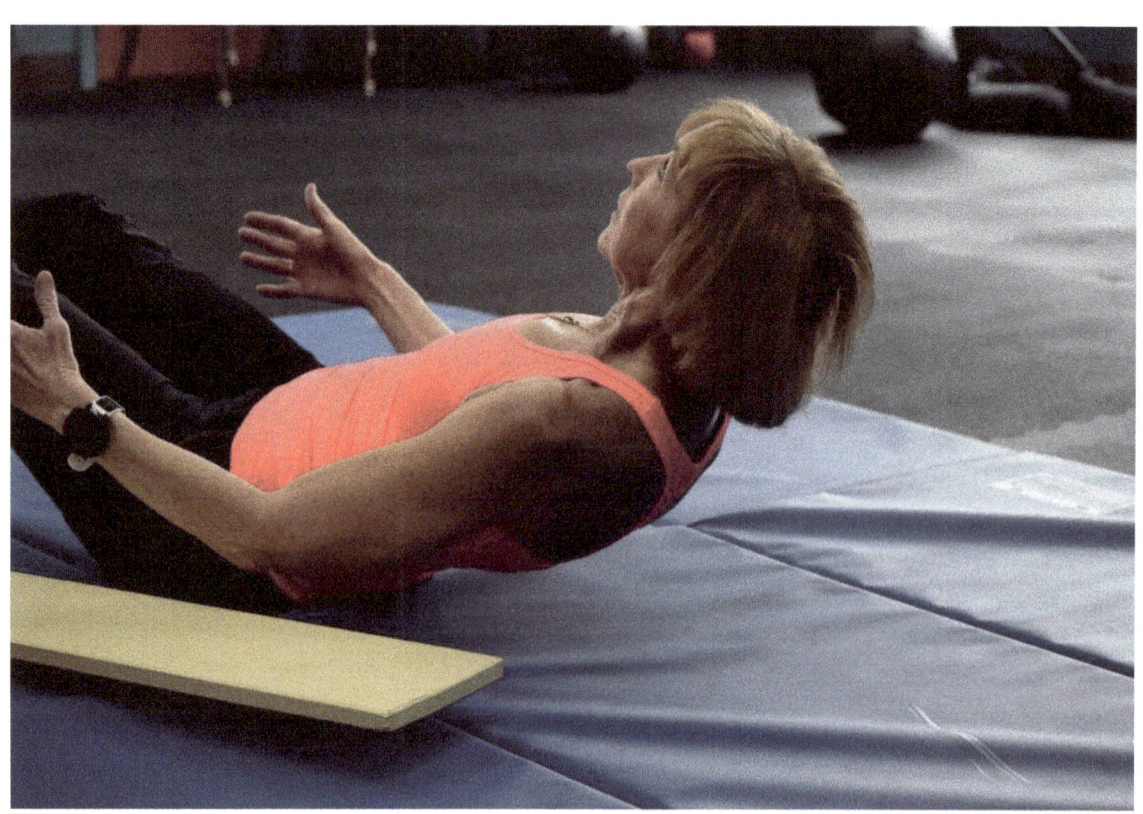

Concepts That Protect

A *Safer Fall* backwards starts by dropping your chin to your chest. **(Priority One, protect the head.)** As you recognize the motion is backwards, your knees should bend and your buttocks should push toward the ground. At the same time your back should round, with your shoulders pulling towards the center of your chest. When your buttocks and lower back come in contact with the ground, your arms/hands should swing back as close to shoulder height as your body allows, to slap the ground. This provides a slight braking action for the fall forces. **(Priority Two, don't try to stop the fall or fight against the energy of the fall.)** Slapping the ground with your hands will not stop the fall. Allow the force to bring your hips and legs up towards your chest, and if necessary complete a back roll to your stomach. **(Priority Three, relax the body and roll.)**

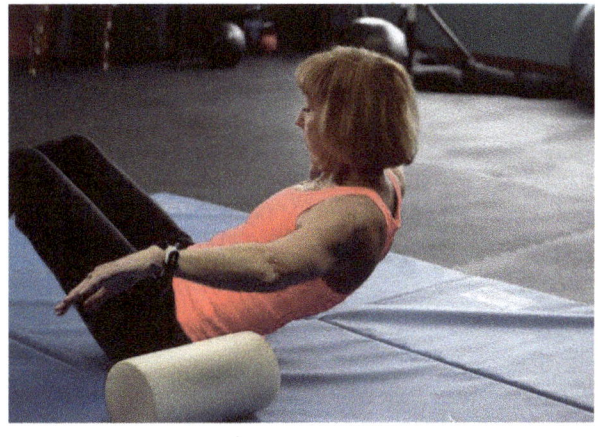

How to Practice

To develop this *Safer Fall*, start by laying flat on a mat or the floor. Bring your hands together above your chest and roll your chin to your chest.

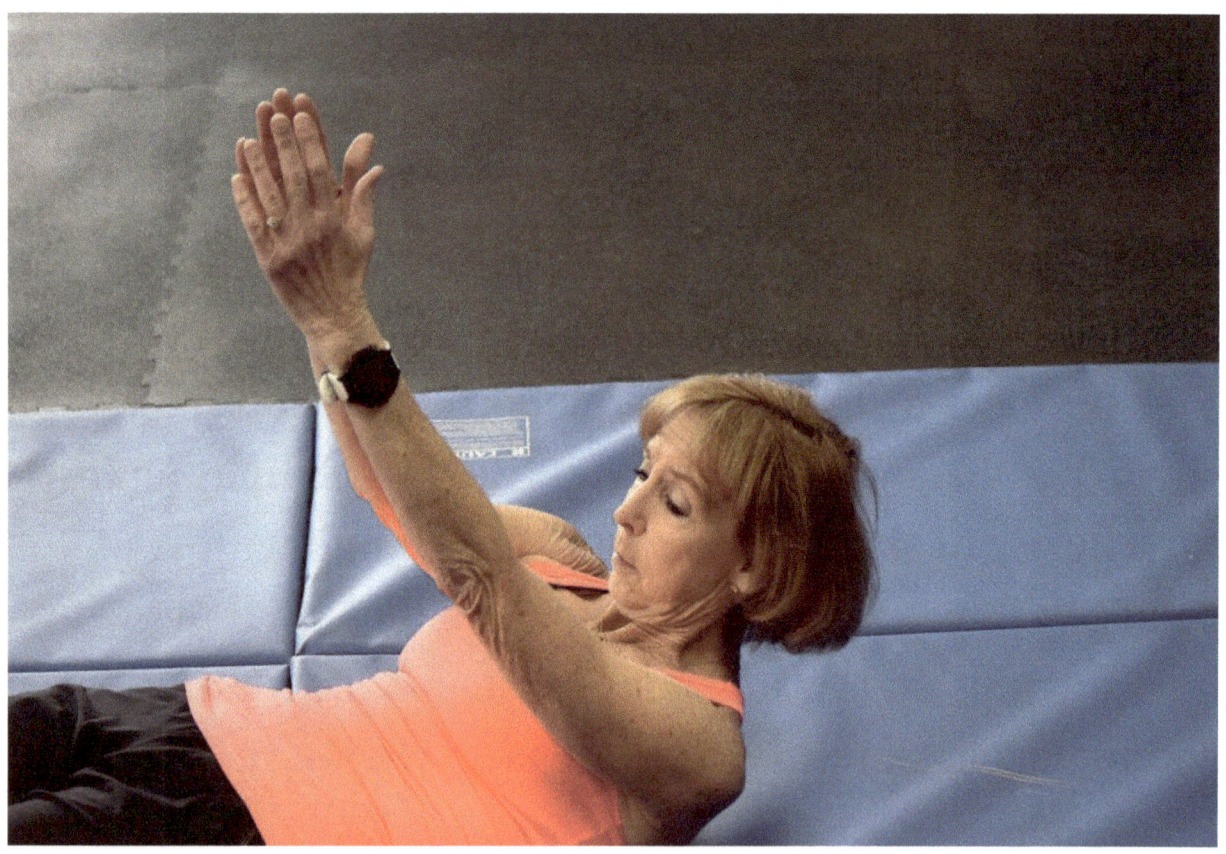

Now slap the floor with your palms down, striking as close to shoulder height as is comfortable for your body. Remember to keep your head pulled toward your chest.

Repeat this drill until your shoulder blades also roll off the ground when your palms hit.

The next step is to sit on the floor. Your feet are flat on the floor with your knees bent. Drop your chin to your chest and keep your hands in front of you.

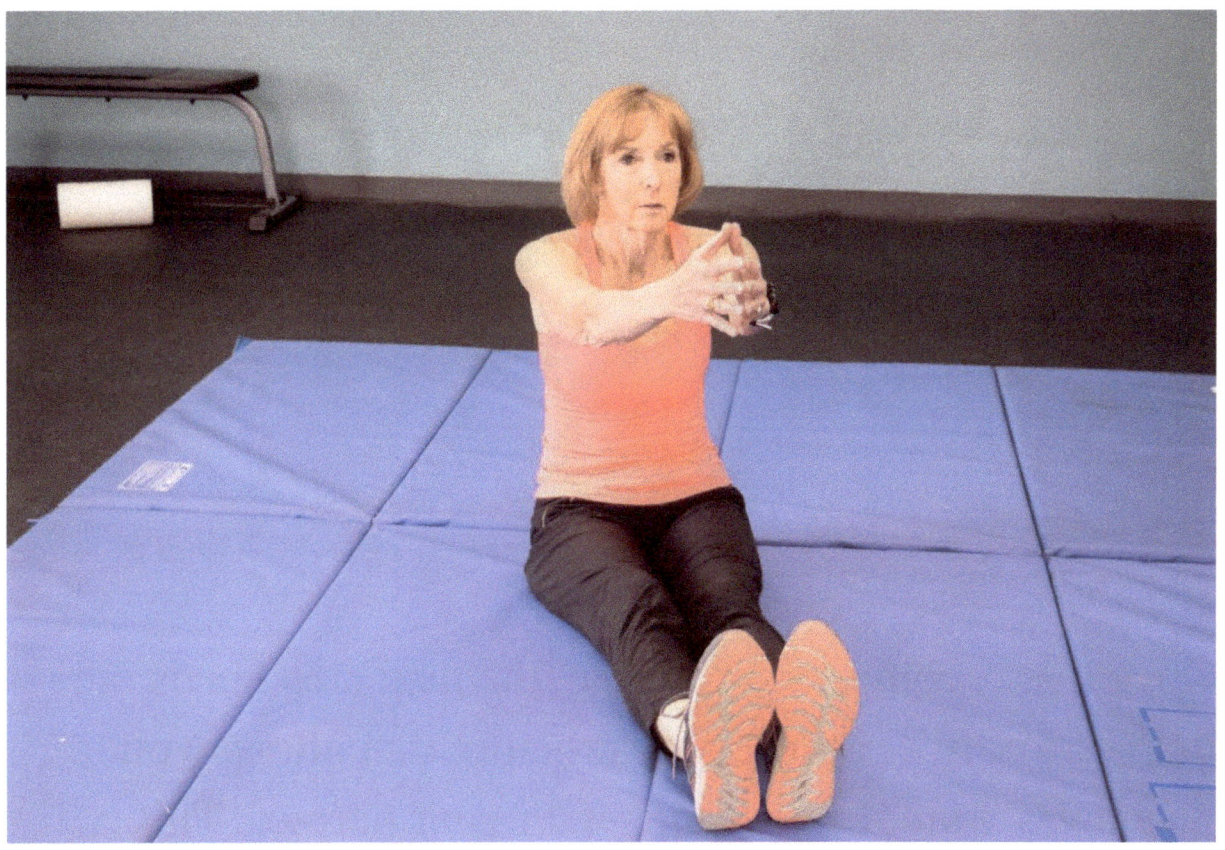

Push back with your feet. Arch your back as you roll on your back. Slap the floor with your hands, palms up when you feel the floor approaching the middle of your back.

Keep the chin tucked. Complete this drill by pulling your knees toward your chest and rocking your body.

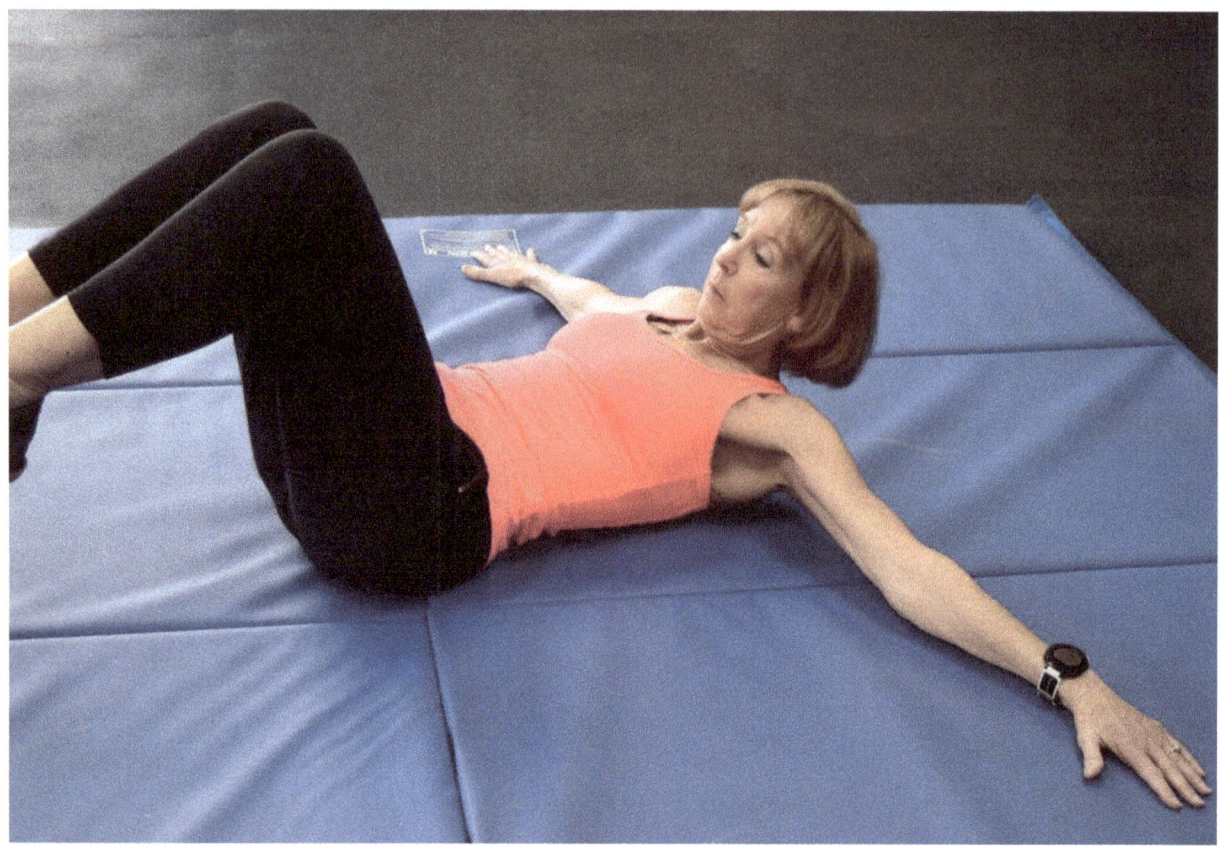

Once this becomes comfortable, the next step needs the help of a partner or a secure structure that allows you to lean away from. Clasp hands with your partner. This will be discussed further in the book. Your partner is supporting your weight as you squat towards the floor so your buttocks are inches above the floor. Your partner opens their hands while you still hold on.

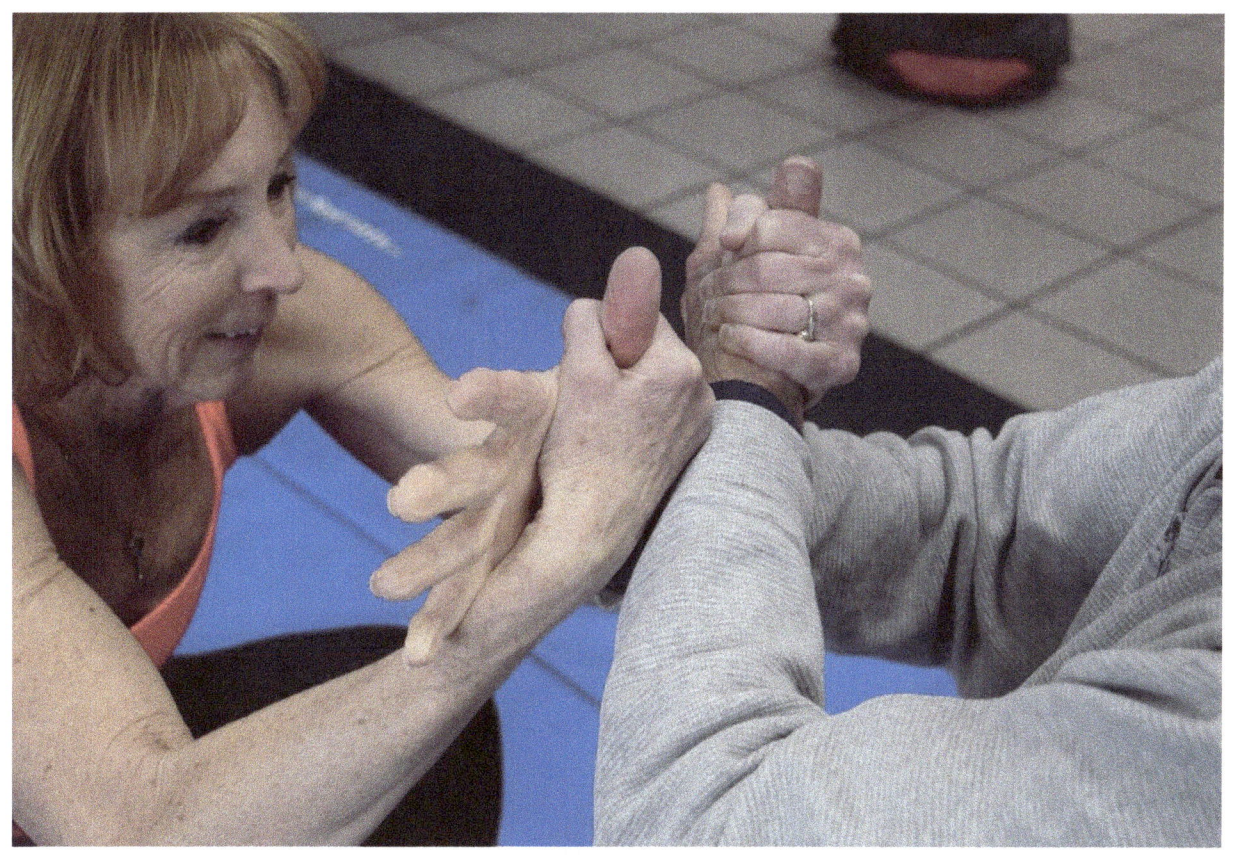

Begin by visualizing a successful fall in your mind. While holding onto your partner's hands, release your hands and lean back to start the fall. Bring your chin down to your chest. Push back with your buttocks so it hits the floor first. Arch your back and roll toward your shoulders. Once the floor comes in contact with the small of your back, slap the floor with your hands hard, palms down. Keep your chin tucked to your chest. Let your knees/legs come towards your chest and settle once the energy has dissipated.

Increase the height of the buttocks above the floor once the exercise gets easier.

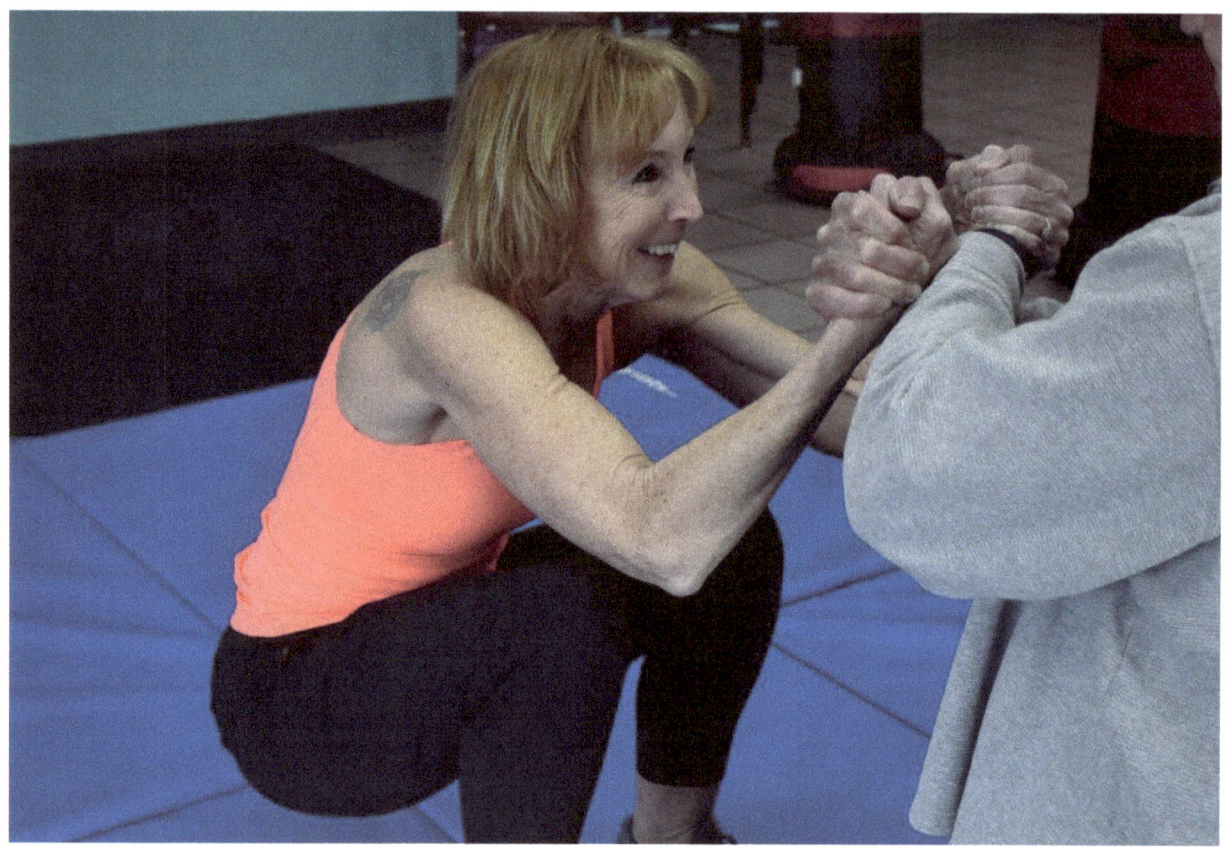

Doing multiple repetitions of these drills allows the mind to rehearse a dangerous fall. Ideally, your knees bend and the buttock is pushed back and toward the floor. Your back starts to arch as your chin drops to your chest. Your hands may search for any item to help arrest the fall, if you are aware of the environment, or your hands are in preparation to slap the ground to help slow down the energy of the fall.

Chapter Three: Side Falls

PLF, parachute landing fall, as the Army Airborne would call it. We'll just say it's falling sideways. While we may use a different term to describe the fall, the concepts are similar. Army Airborne have soldiers that are in top physical health. As we get older, we cannot make that same claim. We will not have a 30 foot jump tower but will instead practice with an exercise ball once again.

Danger Areas or Conditions

Over the years of doing Rock Steady Boxing with those who have Parkinson's, we have seen some side falls. Typically it is a person who misjudged where the chair was positioned while sitting down. Initially, the person tries to brace themselves by sticking out an arm, thus injuring the wrist, elbow and/or shoulder. Falling flat on the buttocks jars the spine. Other times while doing lateral movement, a foot may catch and the person falls over sideways, landing stiff and injuring a hip, possibly breaking the hip.

Concepts That Protect

The concept for falling sideways is to extend the time of physical contact during the fall. We do not want all the kinetic energy focus in one area of the body during landing. We want to extend the time to disperse the energy over as large an area on the body as possible.

When a soldier performs a PLF, the feet touch the ground, they roll to the calves of the legs while keeping the knees together, then to the thighs, buttocks, the pull-up muscles (lats), and roll over the shoulder while the hands are in front of the body from the flaring of the parachute. The practice of this landing is first done off a bench, shoulder height, into a sand/gravel pit, then progressing higher until practice is done off the tower.

How to Practice

Our practice will be done off an exercise ball onto a mat. This lateral movement is hard on knees and backs. Anyone with knee replacements or temperamental backs should observe or at most practice at the shortest heights possible.

Dynamic falls we experience will not allow us to prepare for the landing. We will not have our feet or knees together at the start. Sit atop the exercise ball to the side you wish to practice the fall. Lean slightly in that direction and roll off the ball. Think calf, thigh, pull-up muscle impacting the mat in that order, with the ground side arm slapping the ground, palm down while the other hand protects the head. If you still have kinetic energy left, roll diagonally across the back to the opposite shoulder.

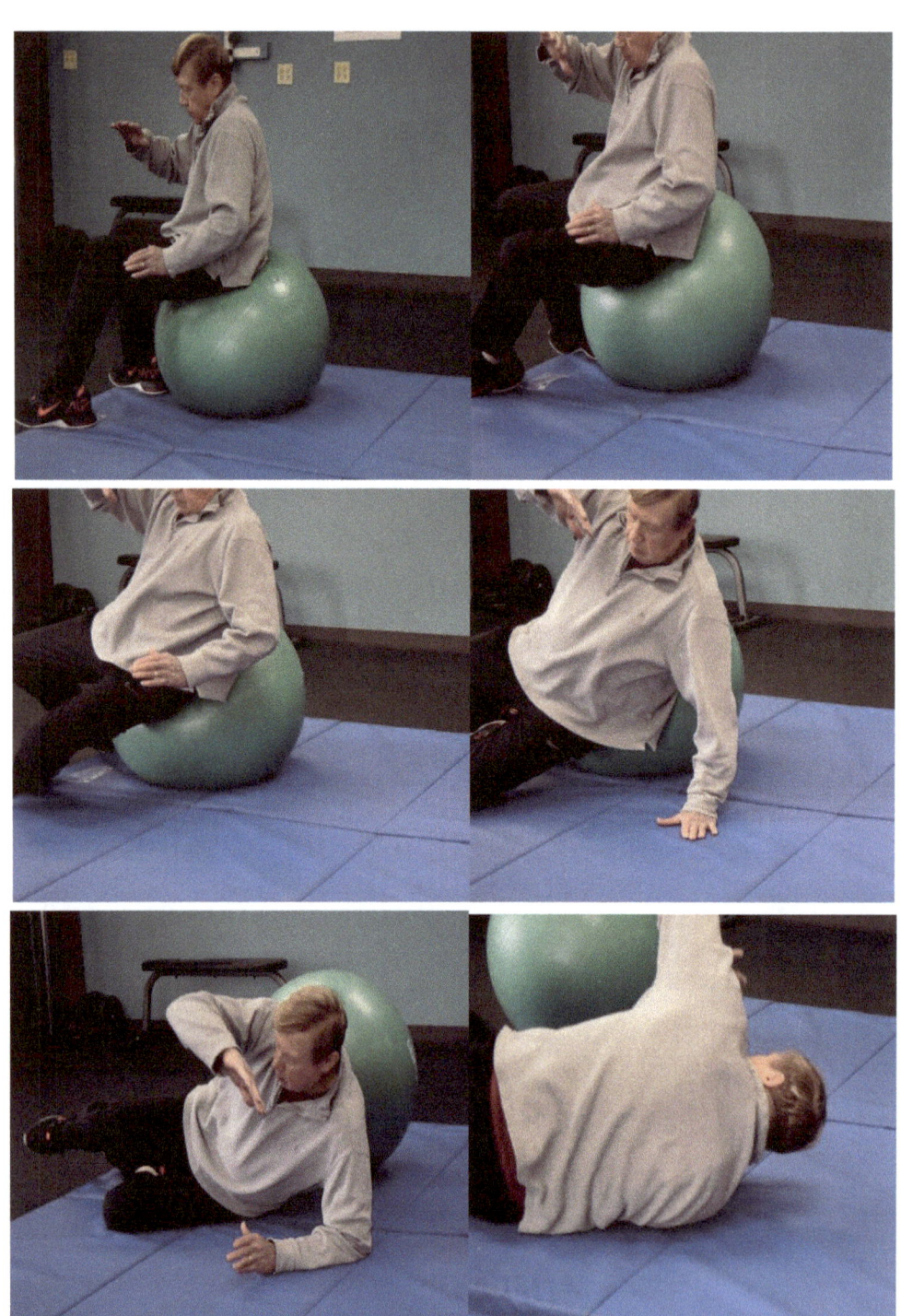

This landing to the side is more of a corkscrewing motion instead of the circular motion previously trained. The side landing uses trained concepts from the military. The circular motion of the forward and backward falls are more martial arts based. The concepts of each are shared as our foundation to minimize injury from a fall. They may be changed a bit to fit the realities of what our own physically mature bodies can handle.

Training doesn't have to be done with an exercise ball or at a gym. It can start at home, practicing on the bed. There would be room for falling backwards as well as the lateral rolling.

Backward falls:

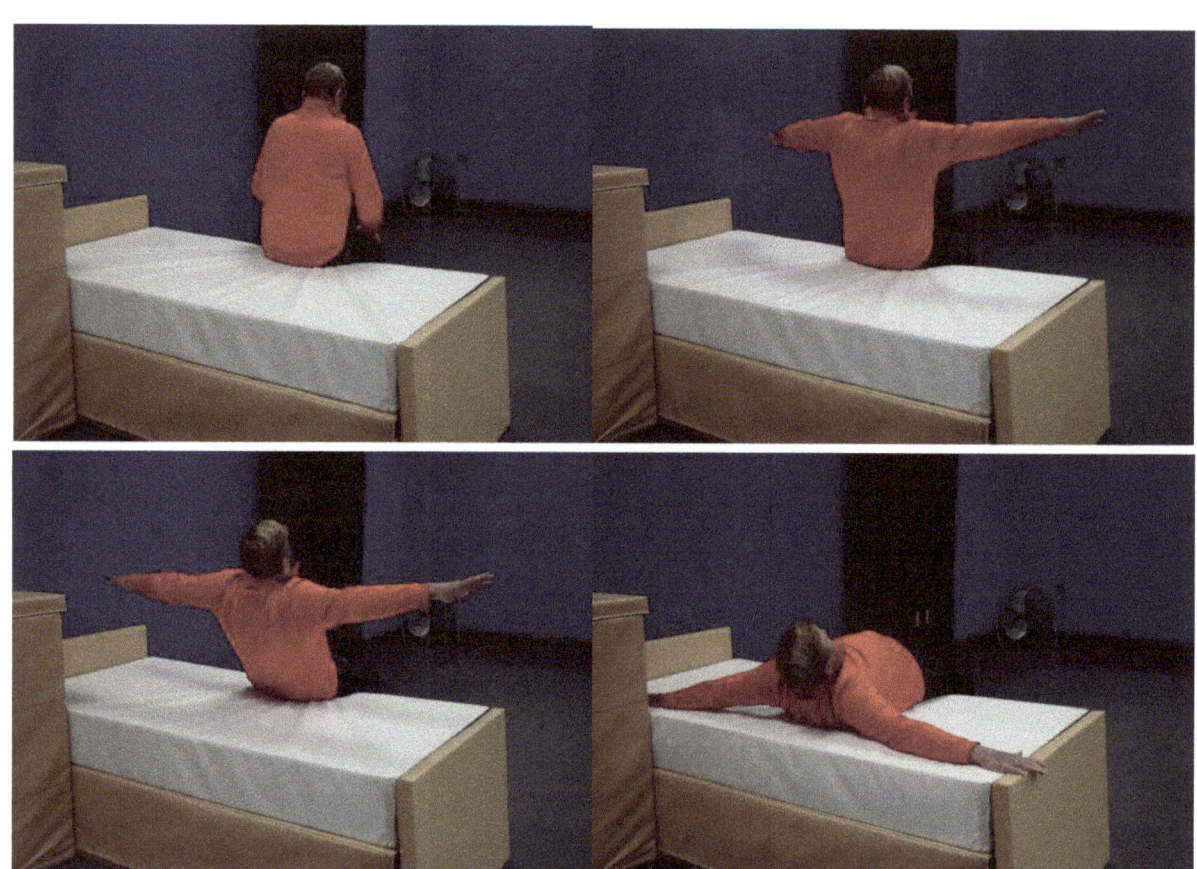

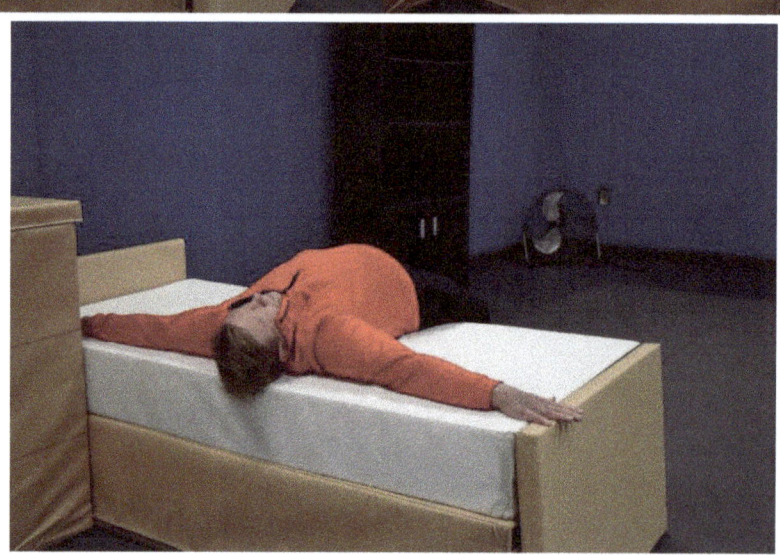

Lateral roll:

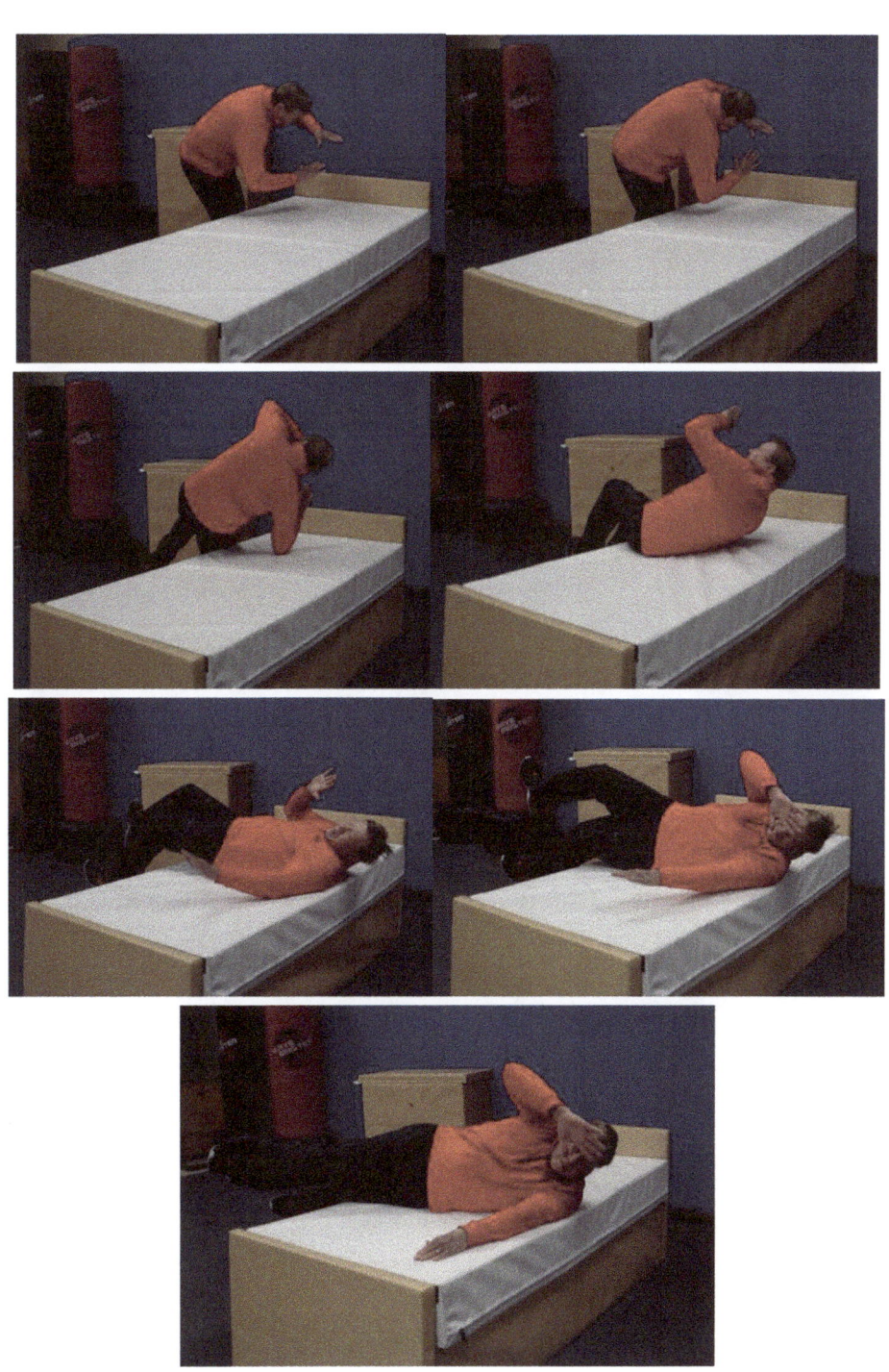

Fall Situations

If you fall to the side near a wall, gain as much contact with that wall as possible. The friction from the wall will slow your forward motion and reduce the energy of the fall. Then use a combination of a forward fall technique and side fall technique. Each fall is different so the safest end result could be a combination of concepts.

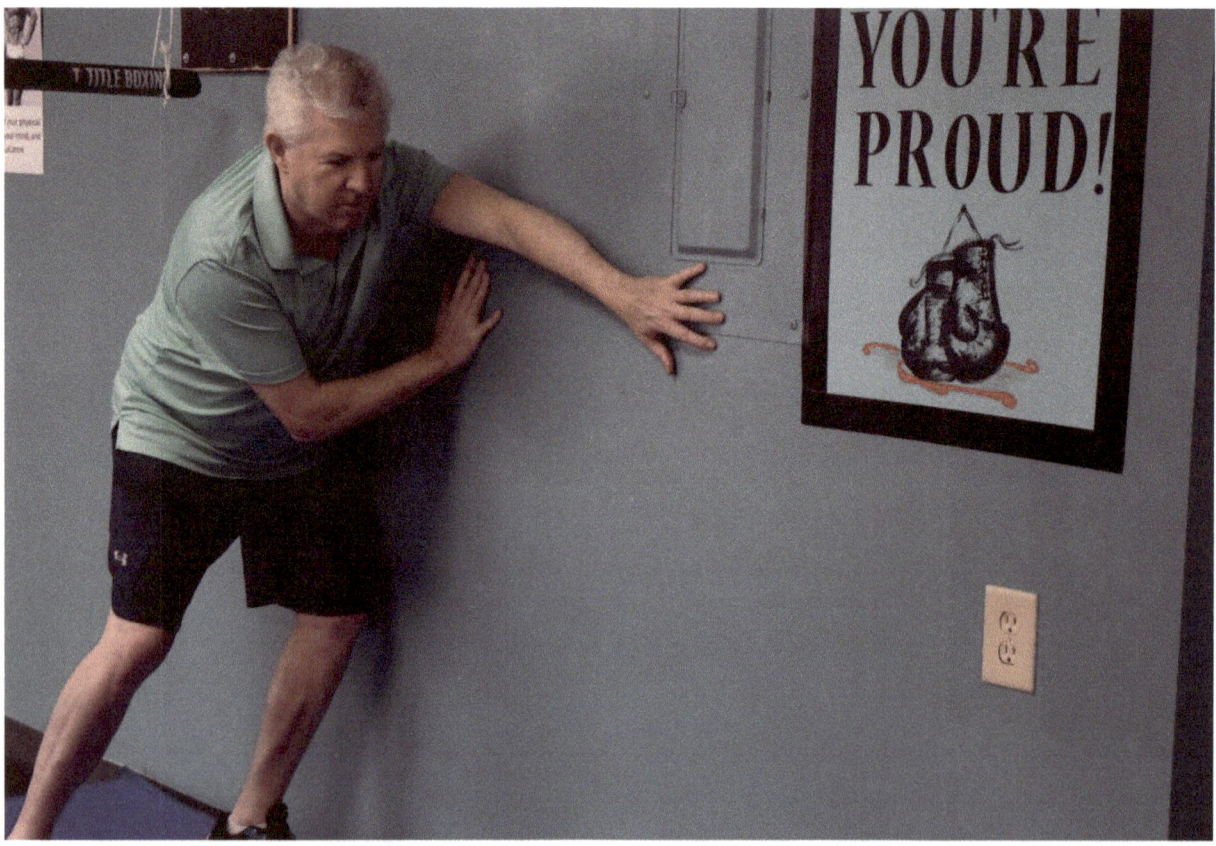

If you find yourself in the most dangerous fall, forward down some stairs, try to remember the priorities of a *Safer Fall*. Protect your head by bringing your chin to your chest. Don't try to stop the fall once it has started. Lean toward the nearest wall. If possible, reach for a handrail; otherwise keep your arms close to protect your head. Roll towards your shoulder and back. Finally, relax and roll until the kinetic energy dissipates. Accept it may hurt (a lot) but the glory (of surviving) lives forever.

Chapter Four: Assist to Rise

If you have fallen safely, the next task is getting up from the ground as safely as possible. The next danger may come from the people wanting to help you up from the floor. That help may be from them grabbing and moving you before you can do any self-assessment for injuries. Slow down the assistance and speak out clearly, if possible.

Start with the basic hand-grip. This is not the typical hand-shake position. We recommend the palm-to-palm, interlocked thumbs position.

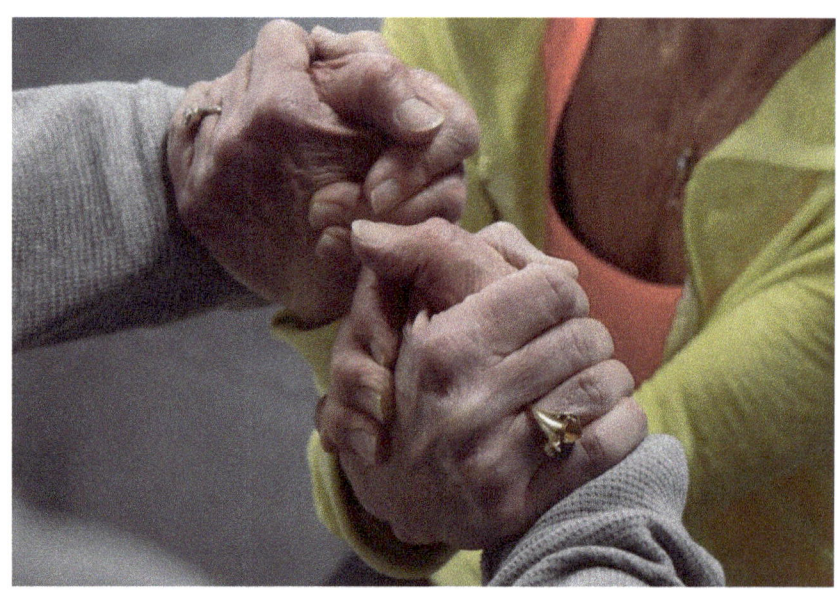

From a Chair
Single Person Assist

If you are assisted from a chair, this grip is the safest and most secure. The person being lifted holds both hands close to their body with the wrists crossed. They hold everything close to their body and try not to move their hands from that position. The lifter straightens their arms, asks the person to be lifted if they are ready, and does a count down. The lifter will use the available leverage to lift the person from the chair.

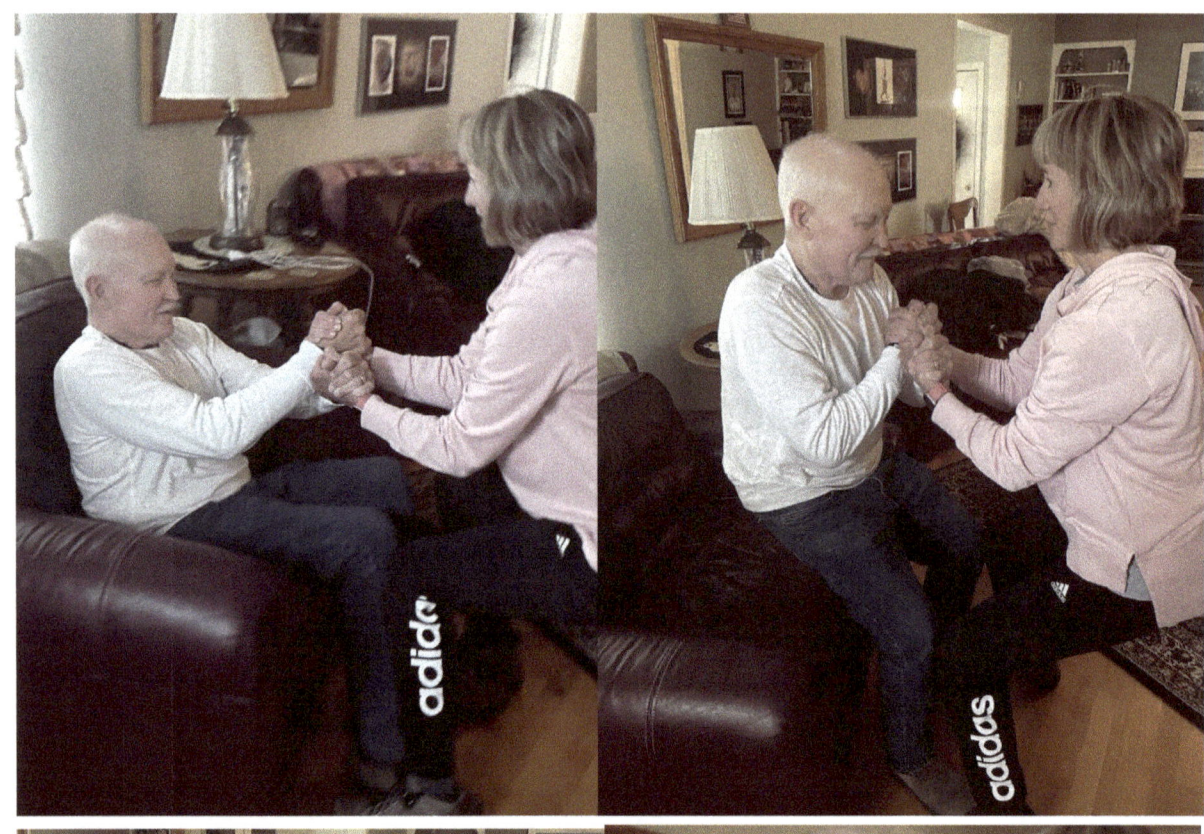

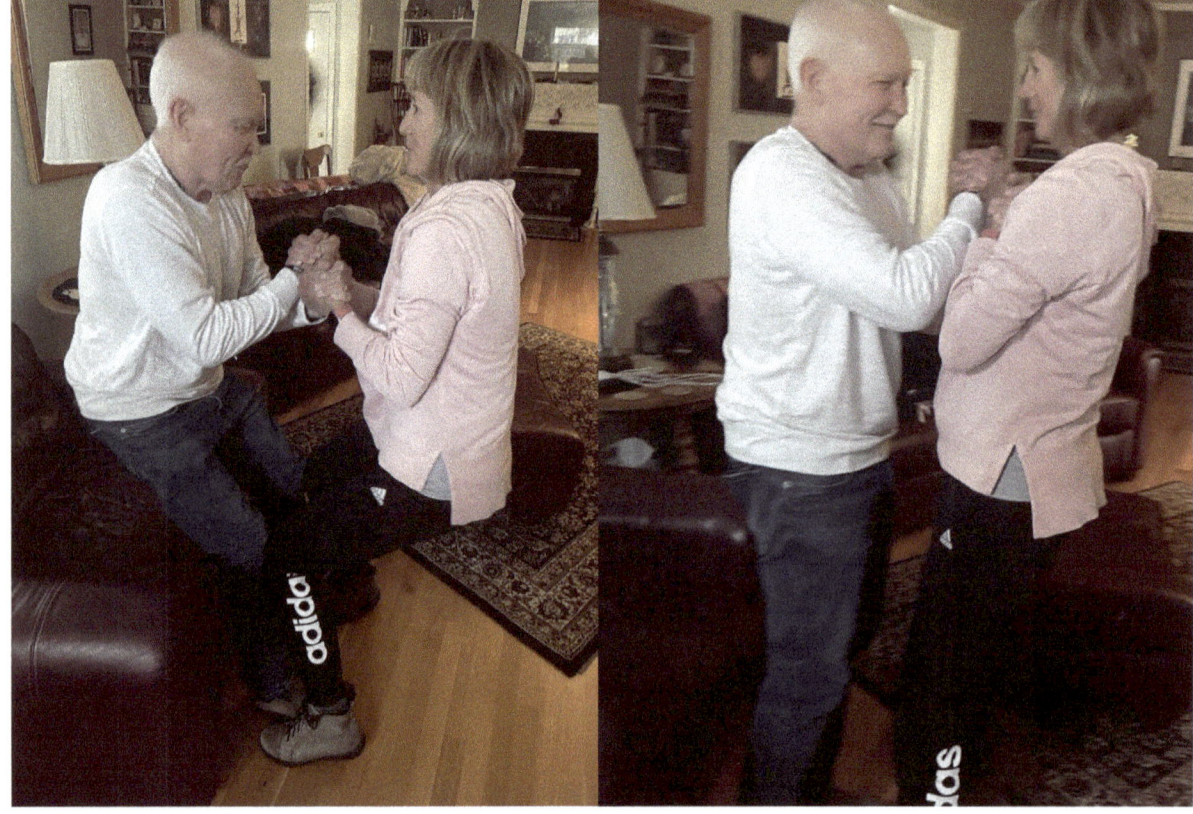

Different tools could be used to assist a person to rise, such lift handles or even a cane. The use of these tools are dependent on the grip strength of both parties. If the grip is lost during the lift, then a fall is possible with even greater injuries.

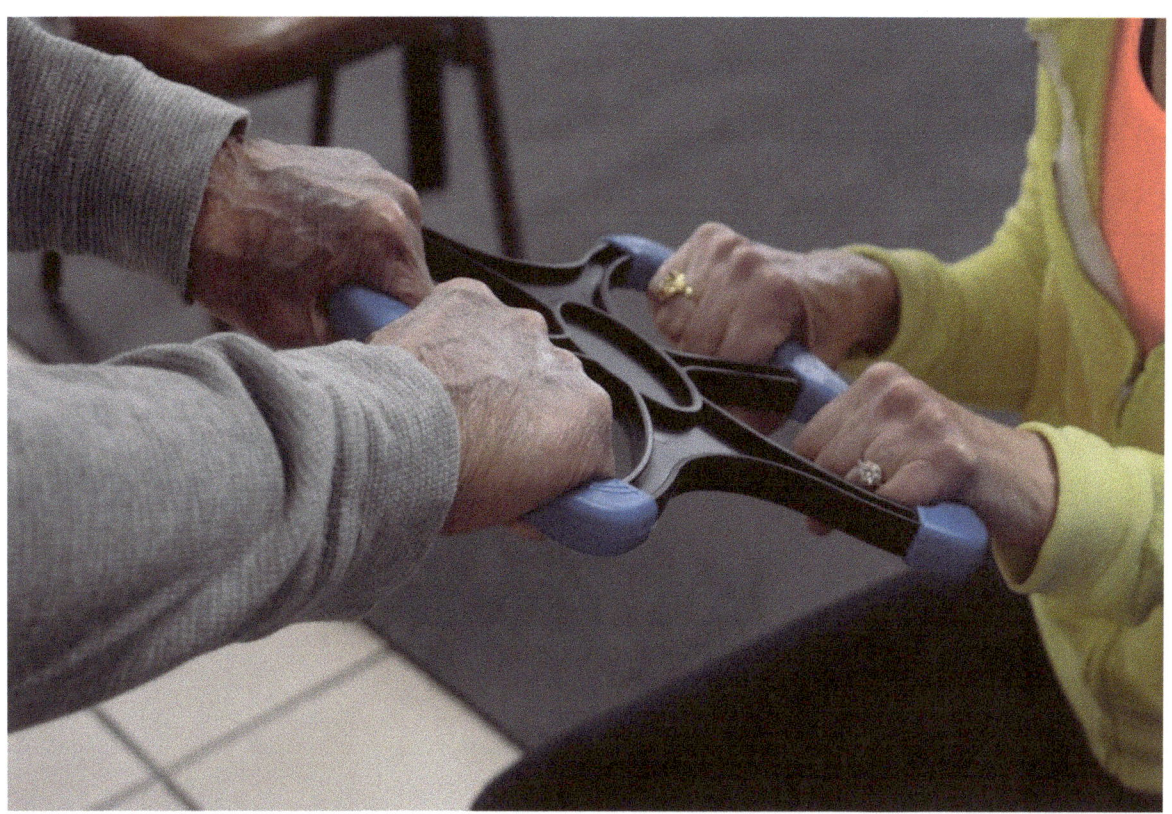

Two Person Assist

If two people are present to assist, one should be on each side of the person being lifted. The lifters face each other with the fallen person between them. They should use the palm-to-palm grip with the person. The lifters will put their back side hand between the body and upper arm of the person and extend their hand until their bicep comes in contact with the body of the person being lifted. That extended hand should be formed into a fist or fingers held tightly together to form a blade. This helps prevent the person being lifted from leaning too far forward and creating balance issues. The person being lifted is told to "lock in" their arms and the lift is started.

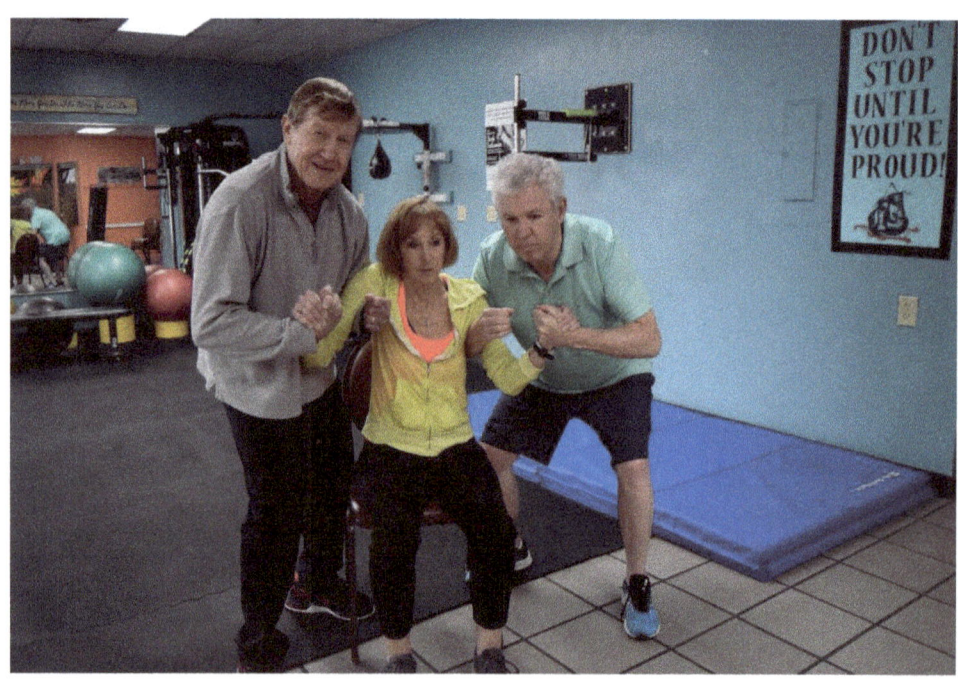

If a gait belt is available and can be put on safely, it has the advantage of lifting at a lower center of gravity. Some gait belts have hold handles attached to the belt to aid in the position of the lift.

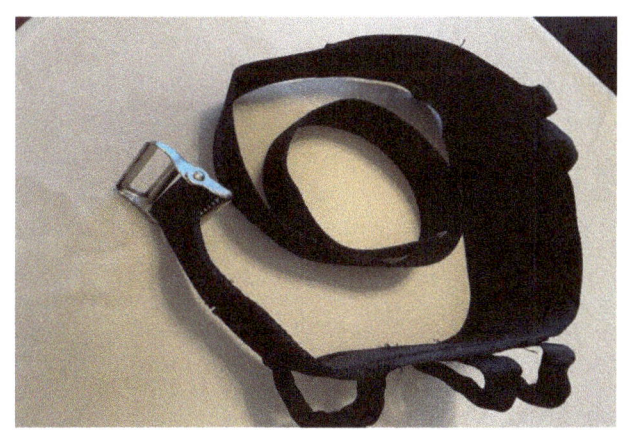

The gait belt should be put on around the waist, not the chest area. It should be a snug fit, tight as it can be.

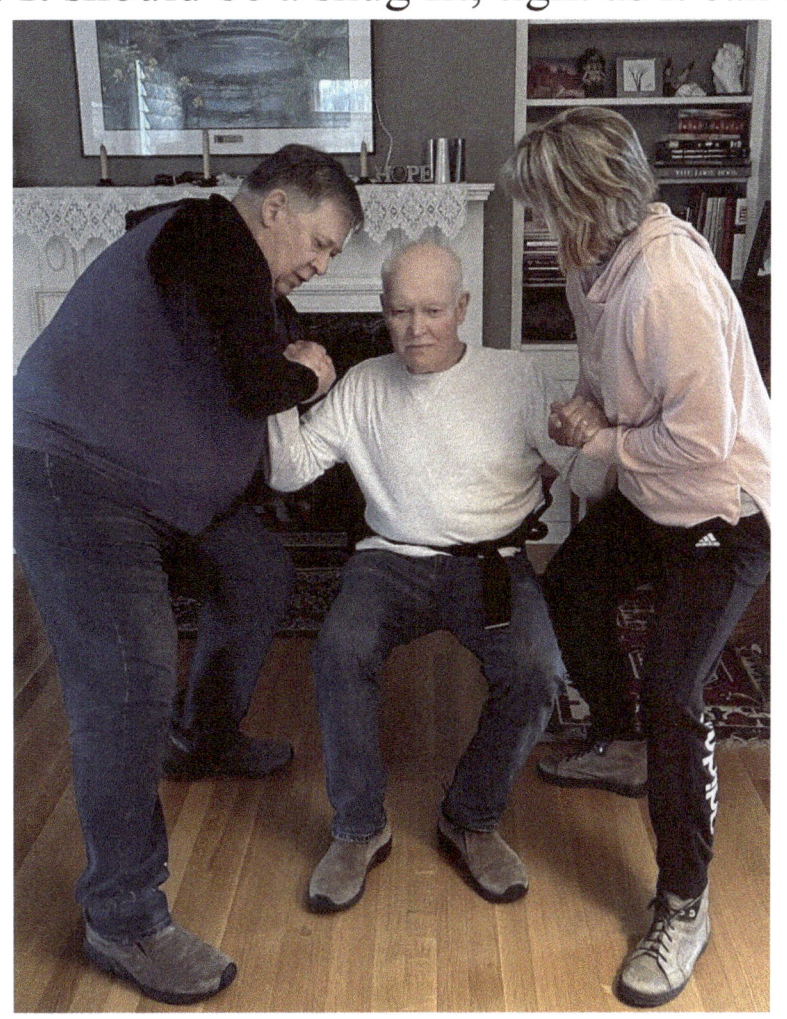

From the Floor

Single Person Assist

If a person is found on the floor, ask if a self-assessment has been done. If there are no issues, ask if the person can sit up. If they say yes, assist them to an upright position.

Move behind the person and get into a wide stance squat. Slip your arms between the body and upper arm of the person. Reach through and grasp the forearms of the person being lifted.

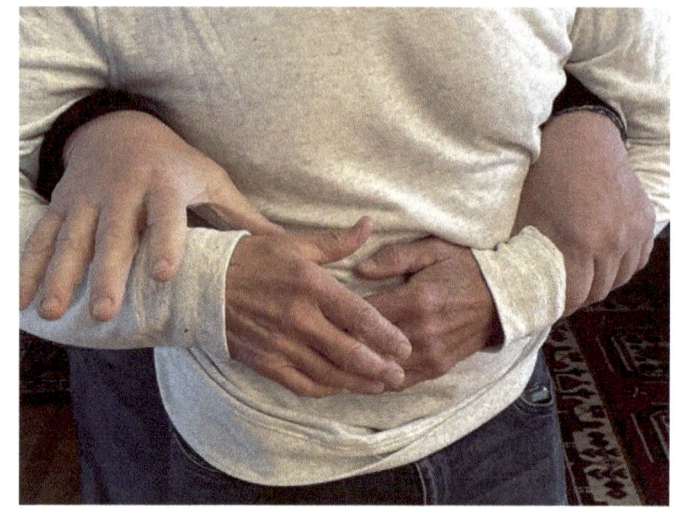

Pull the person close to you and lift with the legs as best you can. Keep the grip of the forearms even after the person is on their feet. Their balance may not have returned and they will need a few moments.

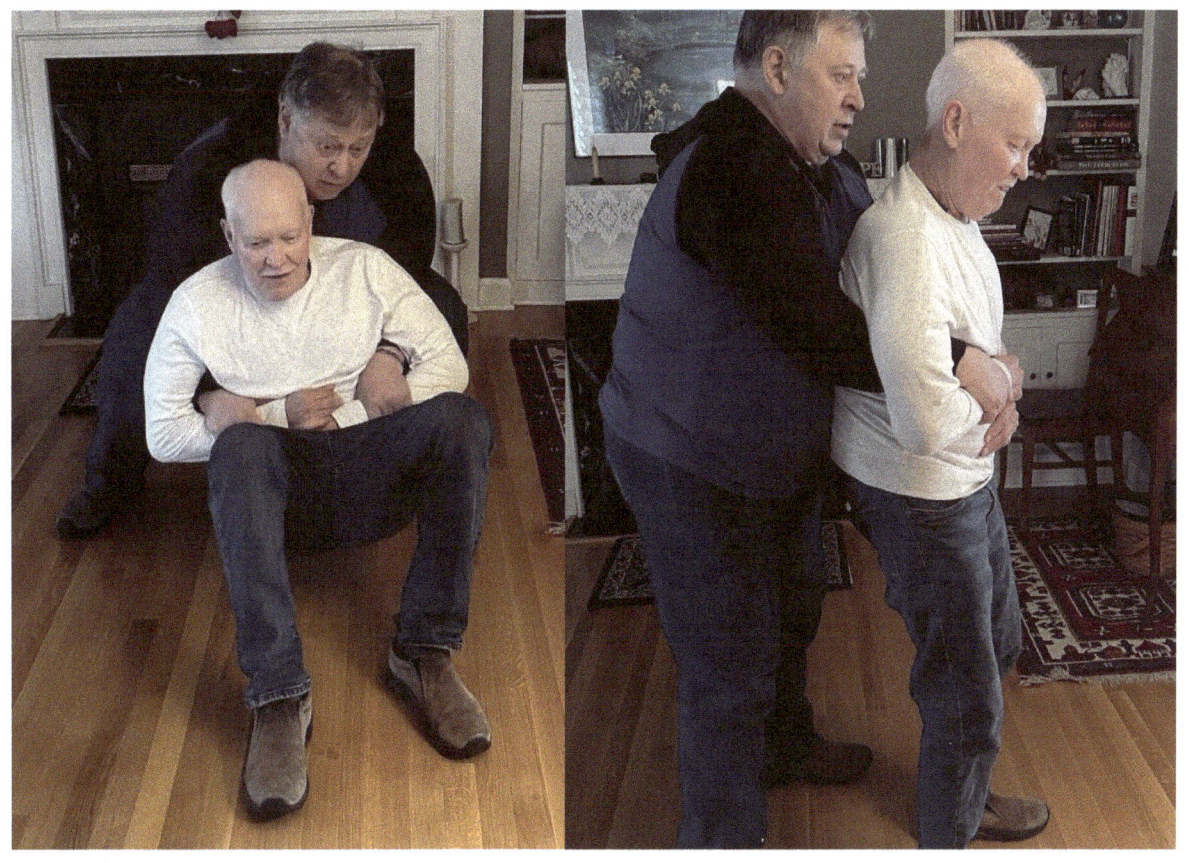

This lift is better than the simple "bear hug." To control the person and get a good hand clasp, the lifter has to squeeze the person tightly. If the person has damaged ribs, this may cause further damage. If at some point the lifter loses their grip, the person may end up on the ground again. With the recommended technique, if a hand comes off the forearm, it can catch the armpit for the next hold. The other hand still remains secure on the other forearm. If both hands come off the forearms, both hands catch under the armpits. Instead of continuing to lift the person to their feet, lean back while lowering the person to the ground. This can be done in a safe and controlled manner instead of the sudden loss of grip.

Two Person Assist

If two people are available to assist in lifting a person off the floor, they can do the same technique as if the person was in a chair, or they could use a combination of tools to help with the lift. One lifter could use the lift-handle and stand in front of the person while the second lifter uses the gait belt. Once the gait belt is on and secure, the lifter takes a wide stance squat behind the person and grabs the gait belt. On the command, they lift together and stabilize the person.

Remember the three priorities of *Safer Falls*:

1. Protect the head.
2. Don't try to stop the fall or fight against the energy of the fall.
3. Relax the body and roll. Accept it may hurt (a lot) but the glory (of surviving) lives forever.

Too much caution is bad for you. By avoiding things you fear, you may let yourself in for unhappy consequences. It is usually wiser to stand up to a scary-seeming experience and walk right into it, risking the bruises and hard knocks. You are likely to find it is not as tough as you had thought. Or you may find it plenty tough, but also discover you have what it takes to handle it.

- Norman Vincent Peale

We may encounter many defeats but we must not be defeated. In fact, it may be necessary to encounter the defeats, so you can know who you are, what you can rise from, how you can still come out of it.

- Maya Angelou

Though much is taken, much abides; and though
We are not now that strength which in old days
Moved earth and heaven, that which we are, we are -
One equal temper of heroic hearts
Made weak by time and fate, but strong in will
To strive, to seek, to find, and not to yield.

- Alfred, Lord Tennyson

Acknowledgements

Rock Steady Boxing/Sol Fitness would like to thank Connie Udell, John Ishael, Tim Scholton, Troy Egger, Robin Stauffacher, Dan Stauffacher, Kelsey Stauffacher Doug Anderson, Theodore Anderson, Elizabeth Anderson, and MC Newman for their contributions to the compilation of this book.